AR: 7.5
Pts: 1.0

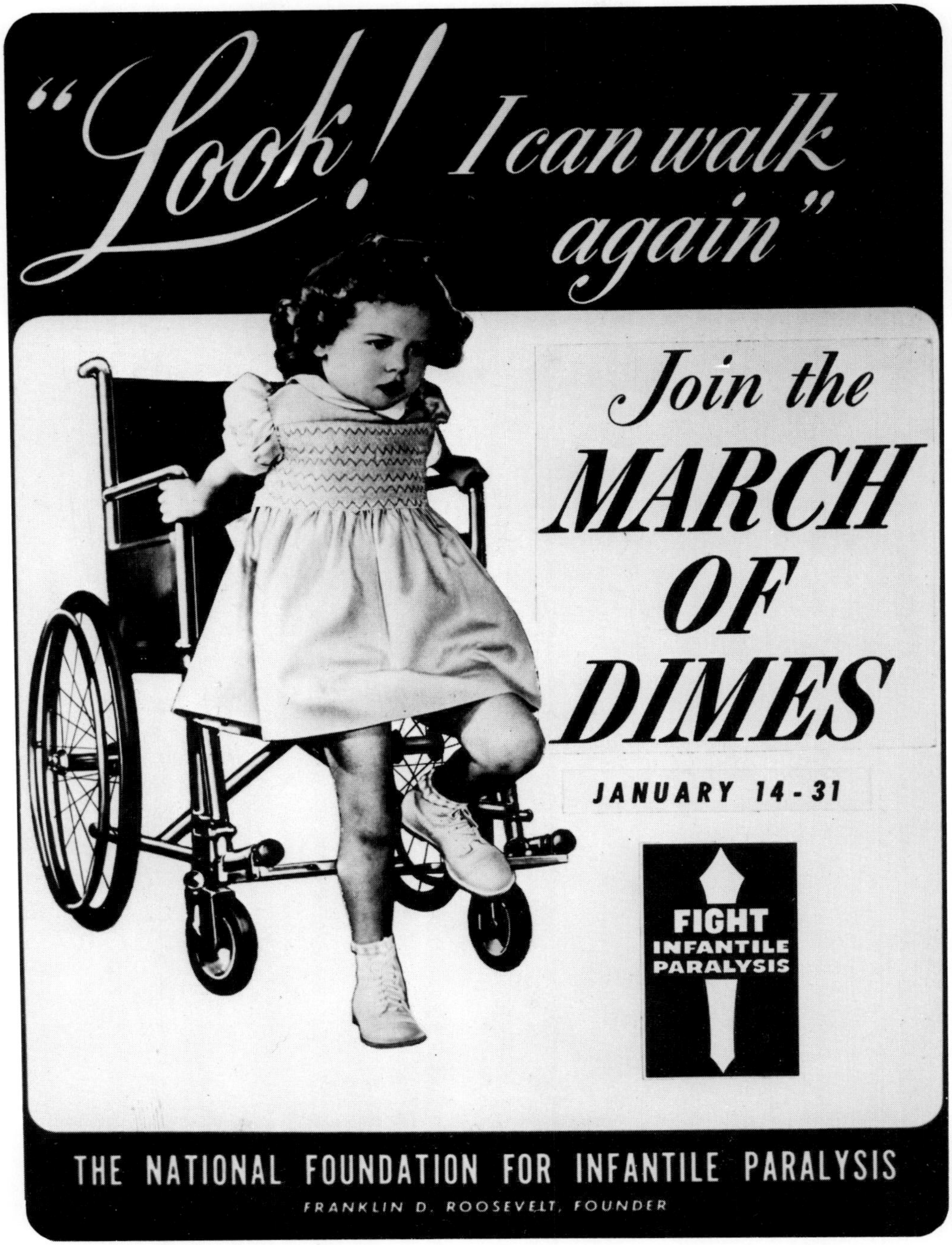
"Look! I can walk again"
Join the
MARCH OF DIMES
JANUARY 14-31
FIGHT INFANTILE PARALYSIS
THE NATIONAL FOUNDATION FOR INFANTILE PARALYSIS
FRANKLIN D. ROOSEVELT, FOUNDER

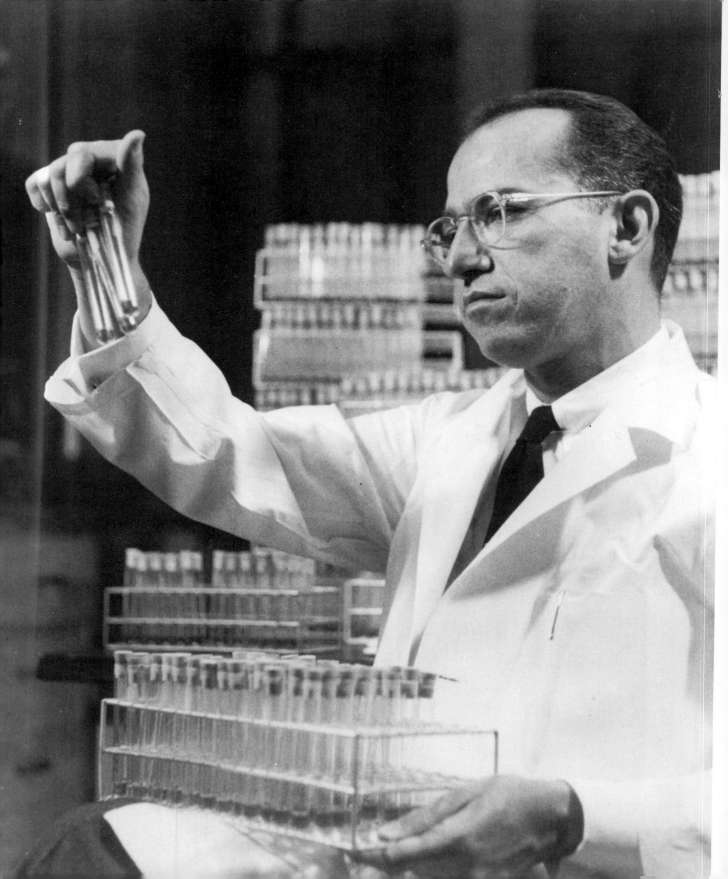

Cornerstones of Freedom

The Story of

JONAS SALK

AND
THE DISCOVERY
OF THE
POLIO VACCINE

By Jim Hargrove

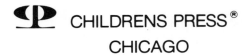
CHILDRENS PRESS®

CHICAGO

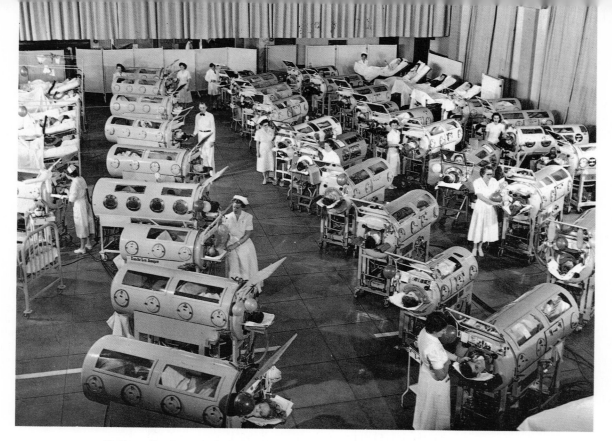

Polio patients were kept alive in breathing machines called iron lungs.

Library of Congress Cataloging-in-Publication Data

Hargrove, Jim.

    The story of Jonas Salk and the discovery of the polio
vaccine / by Jim Hargrove.
       p.   cm. — (Cornerstones of freedom)
    Summary: Recounts the successful search of Jonas Salk
for the vaccine that conquered polio.
    ISBN 0-516-04747-7
    1. Salk, Jonas, 1914- —Juvenile literature.
2. Virologists—United States—Biography—Juvenile
literature. 3. Poliomyelitis vaccine—Juvenile literature.
4. Poliomyelitis—Vaccination—Juvenile literature.
[1. Salk, Jonas, 1914- . 2. Scientists.
3. Poliomyelitis vaccine.] I. Title. II. Series.
QR31.S25H37 1990
610.92—dc20
[B]
[92]   89-25361
                     CIP
                     AC

PHOTO CREDITS

March of Dimes Birth Defects Foundation—
Cover, 1, 2, 4, 6, 7 (2 photos), 8, 10, 12, 14,
  17 (3 photos), 20, 23 (2 photos), 27 (left),
  30 (2 photos), 32 (right)

Wide World Photos—Cover, 5, 19 (2 photos),
  25, 27 (right), 29, 31, 32 (left)

Cover: Dr. Salk

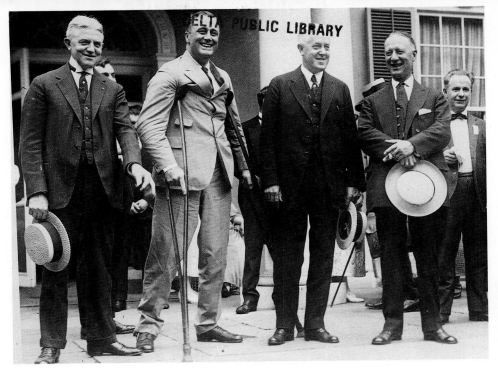

President Franklin D. Roosevelt, second from left, was a polio victim.

Not much is heard today about polio. But before the mid-1950s, when Dr. Jonas Salk found a way to prevent poliomyelitis, polio was a terrifying disease. In the early 1950s, as many as thirty thousand people or more were infected by the poliovirus each year in the United States alone. Other developed countries were hit hard as well. From 1951 to 1955, cases averaged about 4,000 per year in Great Britain; 1,500 in Sweden; and 2,000 in Australia. Although many polio victims eventually recovered entirely, all too many died. Even more were left paralyzed, unable to use their legs or other parts of their bodies.

Franklin Delano Roosevelt, who later became the thirty-second president of the United States, was stricken by polio in August 1921. For the rest of his life, he was unable to walk without help. Many other famous people also contracted polio. Among them were the actresses Judy Holliday and Ida Lupino, opera star Marjorie Lawrence, composer Robert Russell Bennett, and television game-show host Bill Cullen. The daughters of U. S. Supreme Court Chief Justice Earl Warren and the German-born actress Marlene Dietrich were also polio victims. The daughter of American actress Helen Hayes died of polio just a few years before a vaccine to prevent it was perfected.

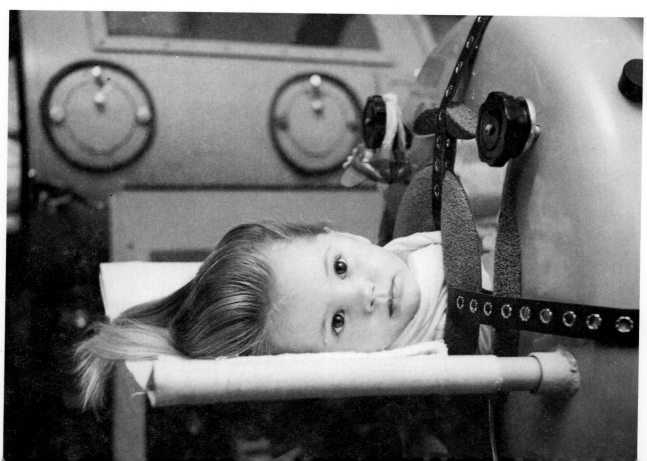

A two-year-old girl in an iron lung. The machine helped the patient breathe when chest muscles were paralyzed.

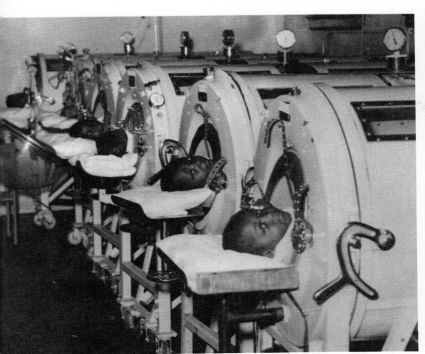
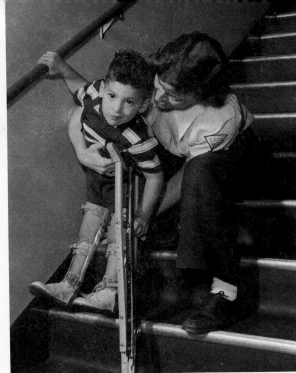

Children were the primary victims of polio. Some patients were able to walk with the aid of leg braces and crutches.

Polio attacked millions of children and adults from every walk of life. The disease was a killer and a crippler. Because it attacked and paralyzed children particularly, the disease was also called infantile paralysis.

Although it is probably an ancient disease, polio was largely unknown in the United States until the mid-1800s. By the early 1900s, it had become a frightening epidemic.

It is not known why polio became more severe in recent times. Scientists have a number of theories to explain it. One involves our increased attention to cleanliness and sanitation in the modern world.

Years ago, before people had sewage systems and indoor plumbing, many people lived in conditions that would be considered filthy today. Germs, including the tiny viruses that cause polio, were everywhere. Some scientists believe that in past centuries nearly everyone caught polio. For some reason, most people recovered, and many were not even aware that they had been ill. Their bodies then developed a natural protection, called *immunity*, from future attacks of the disease.

Jonas Salk, the man who first conquered polio, was born in the New York City borough of Manhattan on October 28, 1914. Less than two years later, during the summer of 1916, the first great polio epidemic struck the United States. At that time, only twenty of the forty-eight states in the United

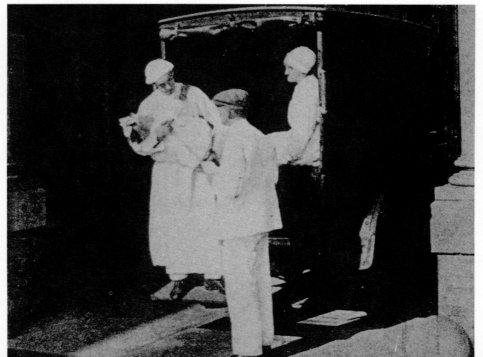

Health-care workers move a polio victim during the 1916 polio epidemic.

States had laws requiring doctors to report polio cases to the government. In those twenty states alone, over 27,000 people were left paralyzed by polio. The epidemic resulted in 7,179 reported deaths, although there were certainly many more. Authorities tried to control the spread of the disease by imposing quarantine measures and travel bans.

The outbreak was most severe in New York City, where 9,023 cases were reported, including 2,448 deaths. From 1916 until the 1950s, nearly every American feared a new outbreak of polio with each new summer. During the worst years, swimming pools, beaches, and summer camps were closed and children were warned to stay away from crowds.

Soon after Jonas Salk was born, his parents moved to the Bronx, another part of New York City. In elementary school, Jonas developed into an excellent student. Later he was graduated from Townsend Harris High School, which was reserved for gifted students.

Jonas continued his education at the College of the City of New York, earning his B.S. degree in 1934. He attained excellent grades while holding part-time jobs as a camp counselor and a laboratory technician. A number of scholarships allowed him to study to become a doctor at the New York University School of Medicine.

In medical school, Jonas Salk surprised many of his fellow students. Most of them hoped to practice medicine by treating patients in hospitals or in private offices. Jonas did not want to practice medicine that way. Instead, he hoped to become a research scientist. He wanted to find cures for diseases by working in a laboratory.

During his first year in medical school, one of his teachers suggested that Jonas take a year off to work in a laboratory. During part of 1935 and 1936, Salk studied independently under a fellowship, a kind of scholarship. He returned to medical school in the fall of 1936. During his studies, Salk learned about several types of germs, including tiny bacteria and the even smaller viruses.

Viruses are the smallest known germs. They cannot be seen even under the most powerful visible-

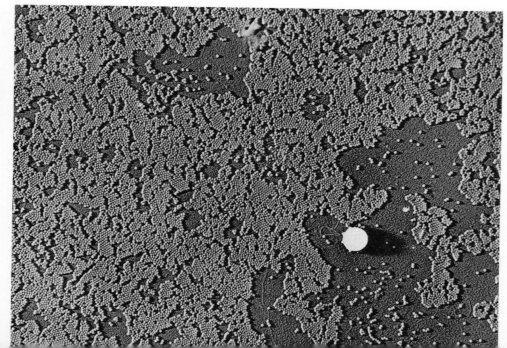

Polioviruses seen under a very powerful electron microscope

light microscope. These tiny germs, however, can cause many serious diseases, including influenza (flu) and polio. (According to recent research, acquired immune deficiency syndrome—AIDS— also seems to be caused by a kind of virus.)

In the past, scientists learned how to prevent a number of deadly diseases caused by bacteria. The spread of typhoid fever, for example, was stopped by vaccinating, or injecting, people with dead typhoid bacteria. The killed germs were no longer capable of multiplying and creating diseases because the vaccination caused the human body to develop tiny natural defenses, called *antibodies*, against them. The antibodies remained in the bloodstream for years, providing protection from typhoid fever.

Killed-bacteria vaccines had been proved effective, but at the time Jonas Salk attended medical school, many doctors believed that a killed-virus vaccine would not be powerful enough to develop long-lasting antibodies in humans. A person who survives an attack by a virus develops antibodies against that particular virus. Only living viruses, it was thought, could stimulate the production of such antibodies. But could a safe live-virus vaccine be developed? If the vaccine contained the weakened but still living virus, the vaccine might cause the disease it was meant to prevent.

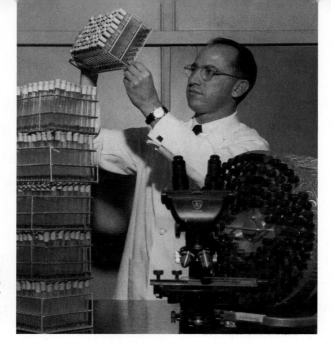

Dr. Jonas Salk
working in his
laboratory

The study of viral diseases offered other problems. Viruses are *parasites*. A parasite can survive only by invading the living tissue of a plant or animal. Polioviruses, for example, seemed to survive and multiply only inside the bodies of humans and monkeys. It was difficult to grow any kind of poliovirus for study in the laboratory.

The electron microscope, which can show some details of viruses, did not come into general use until the 1940s, after Salk left medical school. At that time, therefore, viruses could not even be seen—let alone measured or even counted. How could diseases caused by these mysterious agents be fought?

In one of his classes, Jonas Salk learned that certain kinds of bacterial poisons could be changed. By soaking the poisons in a chemical called formalin, the substances could be altered to a form that no longer caused disease. And yet, when injected into living beings, the formalin-treated poisons caused antibodies to develop. Even at this early stage in his career, Dr. Jonas Salk began to wonder whether formalin could be used to make certain viruses less dangerous.

Jonas Salk received his medical degree from New York University School of Medicine in June 1939. Soon afterward, Dr. Jonas Salk married a brilliant young psychologist named Donna Lindsay. For two additional years, he was an overworked and poorly paid intern at Mount Sinai Hospital in New York City.

In 1942, while the battles of World War II were raging, Donna and Jonas moved to Michigan. They rented an old farmhouse near Ann Arbor and Jonas began his research at the University of Michigan. For a salary of about forty dollars a week, he began his first work of worldwide importance.

At the time, America's wartime leaders were worried about outbreaks of influenza. That disease, like polio, is caused by viruses. In 1918, near the end of World War I, a flu epidemic killed 850,000 Americans, including about 44,000 soldiers. During World War II, American military leaders worried that another such flu attack could damage the nation's war effort.

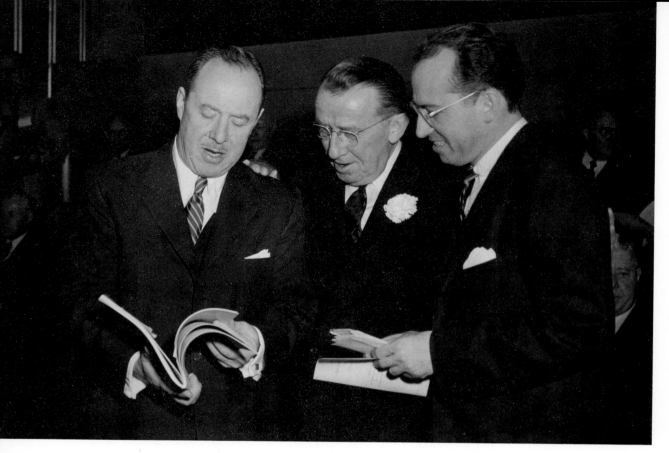

Dr. Thomas Francis (left) and Dr. Jonas Salk (right), with Basil O'Connor, the first president of the March of Dimes

At the University of Michigan, Salk worked under the direction of a specialist in viral diseases named Dr. Thomas Francis. Unlike other researchers, Francis believed that viruses killed by formalin could be used in vaccines. Jonas Salk agreed. Together, the two men developed a vaccine using killed flu viruses that was used successfully in protecting millions of American soldiers. Later, it was given to millions of private citizens as well.

Dr. Salk made a number of other important contributions to the study of viruses. He discovered that the degree of immunity offered by his flu vaccine could be measured by the number of antibodies it produced in the human body. The more antibodies the vaccine produced, the less chance the person had of catching the flu.

His second contribution was perhaps even more important. It was known that there are many kinds of flu, each caused by a different virus. Salk discovered that a single flu vaccine could include a number of different types of killed viruses. Thus, a single injection could help prevent a number of different types of flu. Both discoveries were important for his future work with polio.

Dr. Salk remained at the University of Michigan for 5½ years. Then, against the advice of almost everyone he asked, he decided to join the staff of the University of Pittsburgh School of Medicine in Pennsylvania.

In 1947, the Pittsburgh medical school was not highly regarded. Virtually all the instructors were doctors who taught on campus part-time. Very little independent research was carried on there. The school's entire research budget consisted of an $1,800 grant from the American Society for the Study of High Blood Pressure.

Trying to improve his school, Dean William McEllroy talked Dr. Salk into joining the staff on a full-time basis. He gave Salk the freedom to develop his own virus research laboratory in Pittsburgh. Right next door, he pointed out, was a large city hospital with plenty of unused space. The opportunities for expansion were enormous.

For a short time, Jonas Salk continued his work on flu vaccines in his cramped quarters at the University of Pittsburgh. But he soon decided to change his focus.

A small army of medical researchers and technicians had been waging a losing war against polio for decades. The National Foundation for Infantile Paralysis (NFIP), founded in 1938 by President Franklin D. Roosevelt, helped organize and pay for this research.

For years, the NFIP ran a huge fund-raising program called the March of Dimes. March of Dimes volunteers visited Americans by the millions in their homes, offices, schools, and churches. The army of workers asked for contributions—as little as a dime—to help pay for the battle against polio.

In October of 1946, a professor of anatomy named Harry M. Weaver was named the NFIP's director of research. An intelligent man and a brilliant manager, Weaver brought Jonas Salk and polio research together.

Soon after he took office, Weaver made a careful

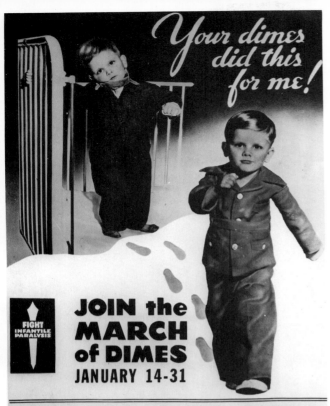

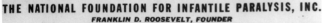

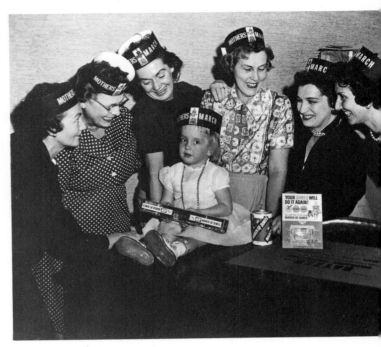

Posters (left) and an army of volunteers (above) were used to raise money for the March of Dimes. President Roosevelt and Basil O'Connor (below) count some of the dimes collected by the organization.

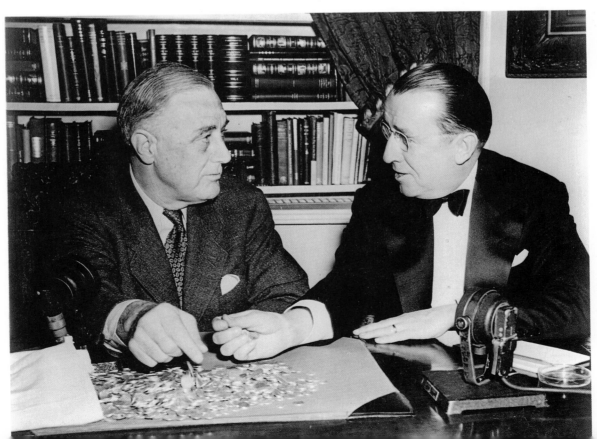

analysis of polio research. He immediately realized that polio was not one but actually several different diseases. He wondered how many kinds of viruses caused the group of diseases called polio. Before polio could be stopped, Dr. Weaver knew, certain things about every kind of virus that caused polio had to be identified and understood.

It was already known that a person who had survived one kind of polio could be attacked by another variety of the disease. Did each type of virus require a specific immunity? Would human antibodies created to fight one virus protect people against certain others? How many? Which ones?

Weaver understood that the answers could be found only by classifying every type of virus capable of causing polio. It was a huge job. Weaver knew about the brilliant work Jonas Salk had performed on influenza viruses. He also knew that Salk was slaving away in cramped quarters at the underfunded University of Pittsburgh medical school.

Harry Weaver traveled to Pittsburgh, Pennsylvania, and held a series of meetings with Jonas Salk, William McEllroy, and other medical researchers. The Pittsburgh team jumped at the opportunity to conduct the virus classification.

By early 1948, Dr. Salk had begun a series of intensive meetings with other brilliant researchers

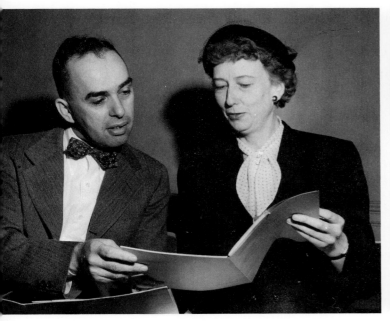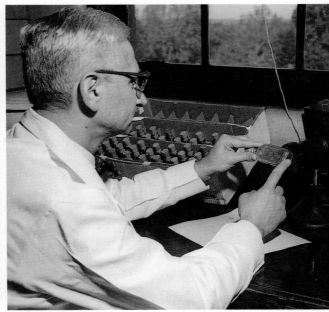

Left: Dr. David Bodian with Dr. Dorothy M. Horstmann of Yale University.
Right: Dr. Albert Sabin examines strains of poliovirus.

in virology. Among the men he met were Dr. David Bodian of Johns Hopkins University in Baltimore and Albert B. Sabin of Cincinnati Children's Hospital. These men, and many others, shared what knowledge they had about polioviruses. By the following year, Dr. Salk had settled into his serious laboratory research.

To study the relationship of various polioviruses, it was necessary to experiment on living subjects. But polio seemed to attack only human beings and monkeys. In order to understand the disease and eventually defeat it, Dr. Salk knew that it would be necessary to sacrifice thousands of monkeys. It was

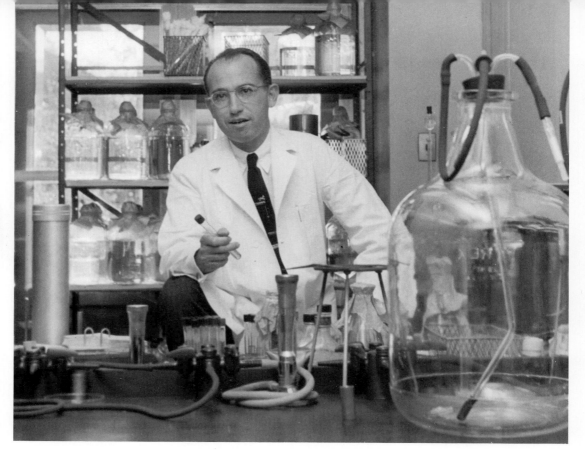

Dr. Salk in his laboratory at the University of Pittsburgh

a painful decision to make, but there was little choice. It was the only way to study the poliovirus.

During Dr. Salk's years of research, the polio epidemics continued to break out during the warm summer months. In especially bad times, as many as eighteen polio victims a day would arrive at Jonas Salk's hospital in Pittsburgh. Many of these polio victims would not leave the hospital alive. Many more would leave paralyzed for life. The tragedy was repeated over and over again, in cities, towns, and villages everywhere.

Faced with this tide of human misery, Jonas Salk

began infecting monkeys with polio. He did so by injecting or feeding the animals with live viruses. Every monkey that survived the illness developed antibodies against a specific type of virus. The surviving monkey was then given another injection, this time with a different strain of poliovirus. If its antibodies prevented the monkey from becoming sick again, it was clear that the two strains of viruses were related. If the monkey fell victim to polio once again, it was obvious that the strains of viruses were of different types.

No one knew how many different strains of poliovirus existed. Nor was it certain into how many types the various strains could be classified. It was up to Jonas Salk to find out.

There were enormous complications. Some strains of virus were more infectious than others. A massive dose of a highly infectious strain might overcome even antibodies expected to defend against it. At the same time, a weak strain, given in too small a dose, might not result in infection, even in an animal without antibodies. Classifications could thus be made incorrectly. Thousands of experiments were needed to end the confusion.

Dr. Salk was forced to spend an enormous amount of his time in a frantic search for monkeys to use in his laboratory. He wrote hundreds of letters and made thousands of phone calls. Eventually, he developed shortcuts in his laboratory procedures that saved both time and monkeys.

Despite every effort, however, he and his associates eventually used 17,500 monkeys in the difficult work. By the fall of 1949, thousands of samples of poliovirus had been given to thousands of different monkeys. Although the work was not finished, Salk was sure he had reached an important conclusion.

Dr. Salk had confirmed the findings of Dr. David Bodian that there were many different strains of poliovirus, but they all fell into only three types. In order to provide immunity to polio, it was necessary to provide protection against only three different virus strains: one strain from each type.

It was time to think about developing a vaccine.

Working independently, two polio researchers greatly helped Dr. Salk in his search for a safe vaccine. The first was Dr. Isabel Morgan of Johns Hopkins University. While Dr. Salk was infecting monkeys with polio, Dr. Morgan was trying to find a vaccine that would prevent them from catching it. By killing poliovirus with formalin, she created a vaccine that produced polio antibodies in monkeys without infecting them with the disease.

Unfortunately, Dr. Morgan's vaccine could not be used in humans. Like other scientists, Dr. Morgan was able to grow polioviruses only in the nervous tissue of monkeys. In preparing her vaccine, it was not possible to remove all the nervous tissue. Years earlier, it had been shown that many humans are highly allergic to the nervous tissue of animals. Therefore Dr. Morgan's vaccine could not be given to people safely.

Nevertheless, Dr. Morgan's work was extremely important. Most researchers believed that only live, weakened poliovirus could possibly be effective in a vaccine. Dr. Morgan's work, using killed poliovirus, seemed to indicate otherwise.

Another important breakthrough occurred almost immediately. Working in Boston, Dr. John F. Enders reported success growing poliovirus in a test tube

Dr. Isabel Morgan and Dr. John F. Enders did important polio research. The results of their work helped Dr. Salk develop his vaccine.

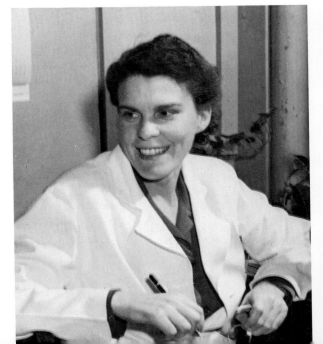
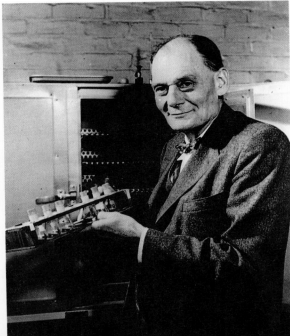

containing nonnervous human tissue. The report was astonishing news for polio researchers. More than a decade earlier, Dr. Albert Sabin had tried to do the same thing in a series of exhaustive laboratory experiments. Unfortunately, Dr. Sabin had the bad luck to choose the one strain of poliovirus that grew only in nervous tissue.

The work of Morgan and Enders opened wide a window of opportunity for Jonas Salk. It had now been proved that killed polioviruses could provide immunity to the disease, at least in monkeys. It had also been shown that viruses for a vaccine could be grown in tissue that would not cause allergic reactions in humans.

On July 12, 1950, Dr. Salk formally asked the NFIP for a large grant to pay for the development of a polio vaccine. The grant was promptly approved. The March of Dimes project had raised millions of dollars from worried Americans. NFIP officials were desperate to find a way to end the death and suffering caused by polio. The following example shows just how desperate they were.

In 1951, a researcher named Dr. William Hammon reported a promising discovery. Gamma globulin, a component of blood, when injected into monkeys, protected them briefly from the paralysis caused by polio. The protection lasted only a month or so.

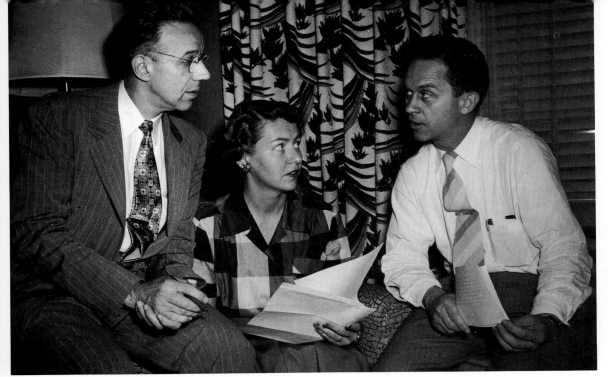

Dr. William Hammond (left) discusses the results of gamma globulin inoculation.

Nevertheless, the NFIP spent $14.5 million to find out whether even this brief protection could be extended to human children. The experiment proved successful and undoubtedly saved a few lives. But it was hardly a lasting way to end the scourge of polio.

It was up to Jonas Salk to find a vaccine that gave prolonged protection. He began by buying large supplies of machinery, glass tubes and bottles, and other equipment that would be needed for the work. As soon as everything was in place, however, a major problem developed. Salk's assistants were unable to duplicate the work of John Enders. In order to proceed, the researchers had to find a way to grow poliovirus in bottles containing nonnervous human tissue.

Dr. Salk soon found the error his assistants had made. Now, various strains of poliovirus could be grown for testing. Then came a stroke of good fortune. In the first batch of tests, three strains of virus were found that grew rapidly in the lab. Each strain was of a different type. Killed and placed in a safe vaccine, the three strains should produce the three different types of antibodies needed to give humans virtually total protection from polio.

The first strain, called Mahoney, was a Type I virus taken from a patient with that name in Ohio. The Type II strain, called MEF-1, had been collected by doctors working with the American Middle East Forces stationed in Egypt during World War II. The Type III Saukett strain came from the body of a paralyzed little boy in Pittsburgh's Municipal Hospital.

Through careful experimentation, Salk and his assistants found ways to grow the dangerous viruses quickly in the lab. Now a great many experiments were needed to produce a vaccine. How much formalin should be added to each flask of virus? How long, and at what temperature, should the mixture be allowed to develop to be sure that the deadly viruses were killed yet still capable of producing antibodies in humans?

By the early months of 1952, Salk and his staff

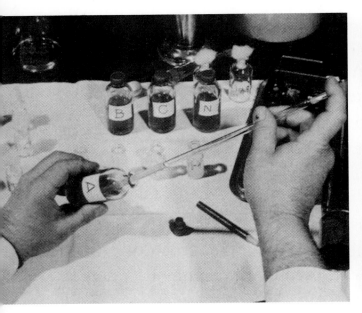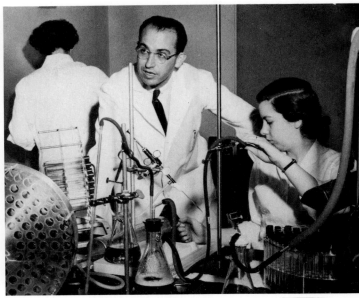

Dr. Salk (right) supervised the making of polio vaccine, testing the different kinds of poliovirus (left).

had found some preliminary answers. The cultured viruses and formalin were combined in a proportion of 250 parts of the tissue-culture fluid to 1 part of formalin. Kept at a temperature of about 34 degrees Fahrenheit (1 degree Celsius), the mixture was allowed to develop for one to three weeks. When the resulting vaccine was injected into monkeys, antibodies were produced and the monkeys had no symptoms of disease.

The basic formula for the Salk vaccine changed, sometimes greatly, over a period of several years. It became clear that there were a number of ways to produce a safe vaccine. In the meantime, Dr. Salk was convinced that his preliminary formula was both safe and effective. After careful study, most members of the NFIP agreed.

On June 12, 1952, Dr. Salk traveled to the Watson Home for Crippled Children, near Pittsburgh. Here, he began a series of careful medical examinations. He found children who already had been stricken by at least one of the three types of polio. These children had antibodies that should protect them from additional attacks by the same type of virus.

A few children who had Type I antibodies were injected with a vaccine containing only killed Type I virus. The same procedure was followed for Type II and Type III antibodies. None of the children injected with these vaccines exhibited any ill effects. Blood tests showed, however, that their levels of antibodies increased dramatically. Soon, injections were given to children without measurable antibodies. None became ill, and all were now protected against at least one type of polio.

"When you inoculate children with a polio vaccine," Dr. Salk told a *New York Times* reporter, "you don't sleep well for two or three months." But for that period and longer, none of the children at the Watson Home became ill from the vaccine. Blood samples showed that their levels of antibodies remained high.

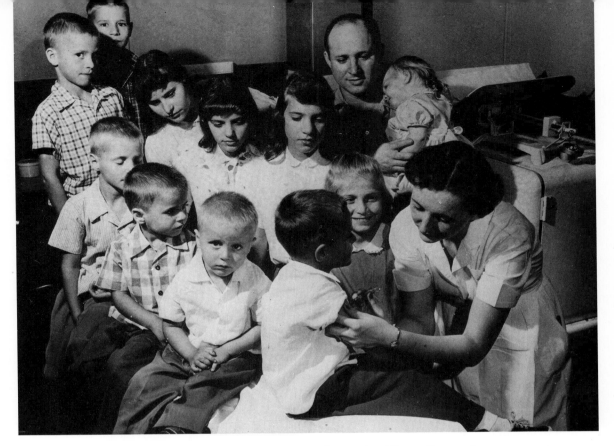
Eleven children of the Bewley family received the polio vaccine.

By 1954, Salk had combined all three types of killed viruses into a single vaccine. He inoculated his entire family, which now included three sons, with the new vaccine.

In 1954, the NFIP, through the March of Dimes, sponsored the final, enormous test of the Salk vaccine. About 1,830,000 schoolchildren were given inoculations that, by the following year, proved the safety and effectiveness of the Salk vaccine. Over the next few years, polio epidemics entirely disappeared from America and much of the world.

Dr. Jonas Salk became a national hero. He received thousands of letters, telegrams, and gifts from a grateful nation. He was nominated for a Nobel prize and received the Congressional Gold Medal.

Newspaper headlines announced the success of Dr. Salk's polio vaccine.

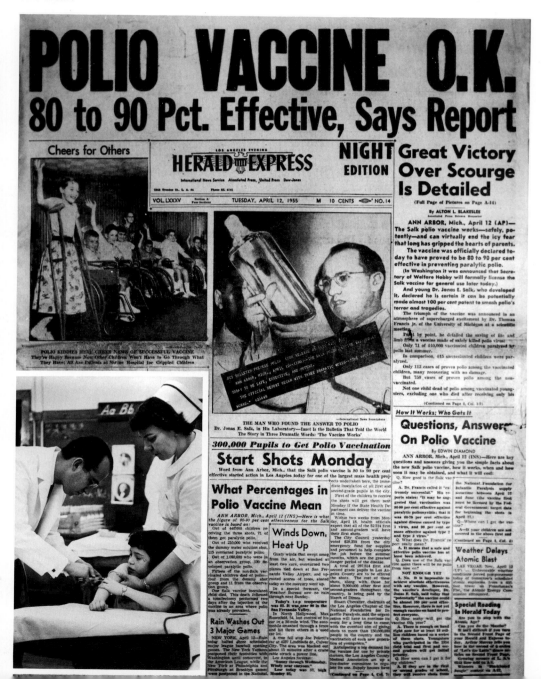

His greatest reward, surely, was the knowledge that he had helped to conquer a dread disease. Although he was offered many high-paying jobs, he decided to continue his independent work in medical research. In 1963, he began directing activities at the Salk Institute for Biological Studies in La Jolla, California. In 1988, he announced that he was concentrating his efforts on AIDS research.

Many people hope that Dr. Jonas Salk has at least one more miracle to perform.

Dr. Jonas Salk at the Salk Institute in 1980

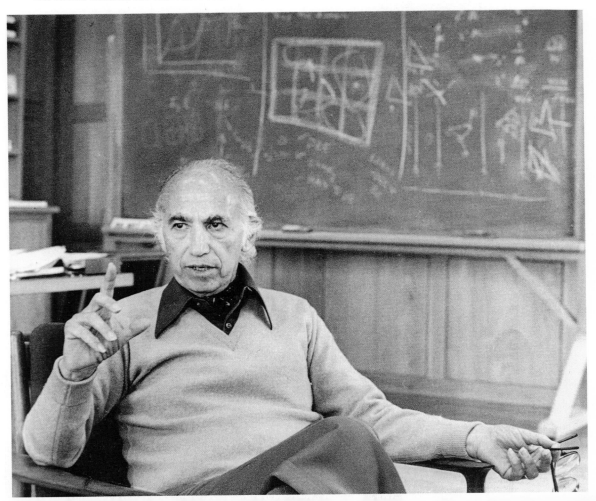

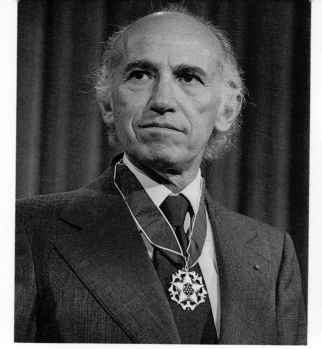
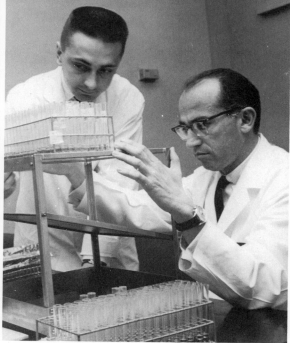

Left: Dr. Salk received the Presidential Medal of Freedom in 1977. The world can never forget the work he did in developing a vaccine against polio.

INDEX

ABOUT THE AUTHOR

Jim Hargrove has worked as a writer and editor for more than ten years. After serving as an editorial director for three Chicago area publishers, he began a career as an independent writer, preparing a series of books for children. He has contributed to works by nearly twenty different publishers. His Childrens Press titles include biographies of Mark Twain and Richard Nixon. With his wife and daughter, he lives in a small Illinois town near the Wisconsin border.